New Mediterranean Diet Recipes for Beginners

Delicious Dishes to Enjoy with Your Family

Summary

Introduction 7

Breakfast & Brunch Recipes 9

    Quinoa Granola 9

    Greek Yogurt With Fresh Berries, Honey And Nuts 13

    Quinoa Bake With Banana 15

    Pear And Mango Smoothie 18

    Cappuccino Muffins 20

    Feta Spinach Egg Cups 23

    Chocolate Almond Butter Dip 26

    Sun Dried Tomatoes, Dill And Feta Omelette Casserole 28

Lunch and Dinner Recipes 31

    Roast Chicken 31

    Chicken Eggplant 35

    Grilled Steak 38

    Beef And Veggie Lasagna 40

    Greek Shrimp And Farro Bowls 45

    Asparagus Salmon Fillets 48

    Grilled Calamari With Berries 50

    Italian Sausage And Veggie Pizza Pasta 53

    Baked Chicken Thighs With Lemon, Olives, And Brussels Sprouts 58

    Slow Cooker Lamb, Herb, And Bean Stew 61

    Holiday Chicken Salad 66

    Costa Brava Chicken 68

    One Skillet Greek Lemon Chicken And Rice 71

Trout With Wilted Greens 77

One Skillet Chicken In Roasted Red Pepper Sauce 79

Mediterranean Minestrone Soup 82

Baked Shrimp Stew 86

Rainbow Salad With Roasted Chickpeas 90

Sour And Sweet Fish 93

Papaya Mangetout Stew 95

Mediterranean Pork Pita Sandwich 97

Salmon With Warm Tomato-olive Salad 101

Sauces and Dressings Recipes 106

Soups and Salads Recipes 109

Creamy Cilantro Lime Coleslaw 109

Snap Pea Salad 112

Spinach And Bacon Salad 115

Desserts Recipes 117

Chia Pudding With Strawberries 119

Meat Recipes 121

Grilled Chicken Salad With Avocado 121

Easy Fall-off-the-bone Ribs 124

Brie-stuffed Meatballs 127

Spicy And Tangy Chicken Drumsticks 130

Italian-style Chicken Meatballs With Parmesan 133

Sides & Appetizers Recipes 137

Baked Mushrooms 141

Mint Tabbouleh 144

Great Mediterranean Diet Recipes 148

Roasted Za'atar Salmon With Peppers And Sweet Potatoes 148

Introduction

This lifestyle, yes because you can call it a lifestyle, is just one of the healthiest in the world.

The Mediterranean food, and 'famous for the prevention of various diseases that affect people of all ages'.

Precisely for this reason I wanted to create this fantastic cookbook, with recipes that I learned years ago and that I still never stop eating.

I want to share my favorite recipes with you, so you can cook them with the whole family, and they will love it.

Trying is believing.

Now let's not waste any time, let's get ready and get started.

Breakfast & Brunch Recipes

Quinoa Granola

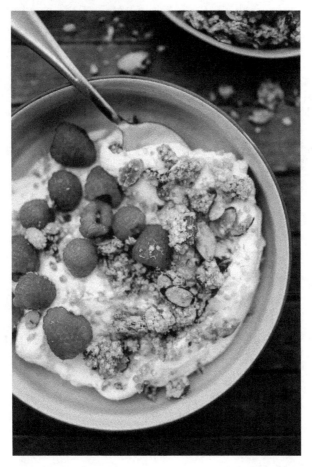

Servings: 2

Cooking Time: 25 Minutes

Ingredients:

- 1 cup Old-Fashioned rolled oats, or gluten-free

- 1/2 cup uncooked white quinoa

- 2 cups raw almonds, roughly chopped

- 1 Tbsp coconut sugar or sub organic brown sugar, muscovado, or organic cane sugar

- 1 pinch sea salt

- 3 1/2 tbsp coconut oil

- 1/4 cup maple syrup or agave nectar

Directions:

1. Preheat oven to 340 degrees F

2. In a large mixing bowl, add the quinoa, almonds, oats, coconut sugar, and salt, stir to combine

3. To a small saucepan, add the maple syrup and coconut oil, warm over medium heat for 2-minutes, whisking frequently until completely mixed and combined

4. Immediately pour over the dry ingredients, stir to combine and thoroughly all oats and nuts

5. Arrange on a large baking sheet, spread into an even layer

6. Bake for 20 minutes

7. Then remove from oven, stir and toss the granola - make sure to turn the pan around so the other end goes into the oven first and bakes

8. evenly

9. Bake for 5-10 minutes more - watch carefully so it doesn't burn and it's golden brown and very fragrant

10. Allow to cool completely, then store in a container for up to 7 days

Nutrition Info:Per Serving: Calories:332;Total Carbohydrates: 30g;Total Fat: 20g;Protein: 9g

Greek Yogurt With Fresh Berries, Honey And Nuts

Servings: 1

Cooking Time: 5 Minutes

Ingredients:

- 6 oz. nonfat plain Greek yogurt

- 1/2 cup fresh berries of your choice

- 1 tbsp .25 oz crushed walnuts

- 1 tbsp honey

Directions:

1. In a jar with a lid, add the yogurt

2. Top with berries and a drizzle of honey

3. Top with the lid and store in the fridge for 2-days

4. To Serve: Add the granola or nuts, enjoy

Nutrition Info:Per Serving: Calories:2;Carbs: 35g;Total Fat: 4g;Protein: 19g

Quinoa Bake With Banana

Servings: 8

Cooking Time: 1 Hour 20 Minutes

Ingredients:

- 3 cups medium over-ripe Bananas, mashed

- 1/4 cup molasses

- 1/4 cup pure maple syrup

- 1 tbsp cinnamon

- 2 tsp raw vanilla extract

- 1 tsp ground ginger

- 1 tsp ground cloves

- 1/2 tsp ground allspice

- 1/2 tsp salt

- 1 cup quinoa, uncooked

- 2 1/2 cups unsweetened vanilla almond milk

- 1/4 cup slivered almonds

Directions:

1. In the bottom of a 2 2-3-quart casserole dish, mix together the mashed banana, maple syrup, cinnamon, vanilla extract, ginger, cloves, allspice, molasses, and salt until well mixed

2. Add in the quinoa, stir until the quinoa is evenly in the banana mixture.

3. Whisk in the almond milk, mix until well combined, cover and refrigerate overnight or bake immediately

4. Heat oven to 350 degrees F

5. Whisk the quinoa mixture making sure it doesn't settle to the bottom

6. Cover the pan with tinfoil and bake until the liquid is absorbed, and the top of the quinoa is set, about 1 hour to 1 hour and 15 mins

7. Turn the oven to high broil, uncover the pan, sprinkle with sliced almonds, and lightly press them into the quinoa

8. Broil until the almonds just turn golden brown, about 2-4 minutes, watching closely, as they burn quickly

9. Allow to cool for 10 minutes then slice the quinoa bake

10. Distribute the quinoa bake among the containers, store in the fridge for 3-4 days

Nutrition Info:Per Serving: Calories:213;Carbs: 41g;Total Fat: 4g;Protein: 5g

Pear And Mango Smoothie

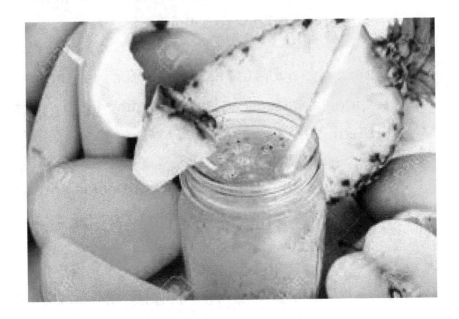

Servings: 1

Cooking Time: 10 Minutes

Ingredients:

- ½ peeled, pitted, and chopped mango

- 2 cubes of ice

- 1 ripe, cored, and chopped pear

- ½ cup of plain Greek yogurt

- 1 cup chopped kale

Directions:

1. In a blender, combine the mango, ice cubes, pear, yogurt, and kale.

2. Blend until the mixture is smooth and thick.

3. Serve and enjoy!

Nutrition Info: calories: 293, fats: 8 grams, carbohydrates: 53 grams, protein: 8 grams.

Cappuccino Muffins

Servings: 2

Cooking Time: 20 Minutes

Ingredients:

- 2 1/3 cups all-purpose flour

- 2 tsp baking powder

- 1 tsp salt

- 1 tsp ground cinnamon

- ¾ cup hot water

- 2 tbsp espresso powder or instant coffee

- 2 eggs

- 1 cup sugar

- ¾ cup vegetable oil

- 1/3 cup mini chocolate chips

- ¼ cup milk

Directions:

1. Preheat oven to 425 degree F

2. In a medium bowl, whisk together the flour, baking powder, salt and cinnamon, set aside

3. In a small bowl, combine the hot water and espresso powder, stir to dissolve, add milk, stir to combine and set aside

4. In a large bowl, whisk together eggs, sugar and oil, slowly add the coffee mixture, and stir to combine Then add in the dry ingredients in thirds, whisking gently until smooth

5. Add in the chocolate chips, stir to combine

6. Place the muffin papers in a 12-cup muffin tin

7. Fill each cup half way

8. Bake for 17-20 minutes, until risen and set

9. Allow to cool completely before slicing

10. Wrap the slices in plastic wrap and then aluminum foil and store in fridge for up to 4-5 days

11. To Serve: Remove the aluminum foil and plastic wrap, and microwave for 2 minutes, then allow to rest for 30 seconds, enjoy!

Nutrition Info:Per Serving:(1 muffin): Calories:201;Carbs: 29g;Total Fat: 8g;Protein: 2g

Feta Spinach Egg Cups

Servings: 4

Cooking Time: 8 Minutes

Ingredients:

- 6 eggs

- 1/4 tsp garlic powder

- 1 tomato, chopped

- 1/4 cup feta cheese, crumbled

- 1 cup spinach, chopped

- 1/2 cup mozzarella cheese, shredded

- Pepper

- salt

Directions:

1. Pour 1/2 cups of water into the instant pot then place steamer rack in the pot.

2. In a bowl, whisk eggs with garlic powder, pepper, and salt.

3. Add remaining ingredients and stir well.

4. Spray four ramekins with cooking spray.

5. Pour egg mixture into the ramekins and place ramekins on top of the rack.

6. Seal pot with lid and cook on high for 8 minutes.

7. Once done, release pressure using quick release. Remove lid.

8. Serve and enjoy.

Nutrition Info: Calories: 134;Fat: 3 g;Carbohydrates: 2 g;Sugar: 1.4 g;Protein: 11 g;Cholesterol: 256 mg

Chocolate Almond Butter Dip

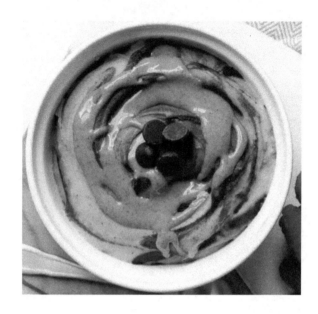

Servings: 5

Cooking Time: 10 Minutes

Ingredients:

- 1 cup of Plain Greek Yogurt

- ½ cup almond butter

- 1/3 cup chocolate hazelnut spread

- 1 tablespoon honey

- 1 teaspoon vanilla

- sliced up fruits as you desire, such as pears, apples, apricots, bananas, etc.

Directions:

1. Take a medium-sized bowl and add all Ingredients: except the fruit.

2. Take an immersion blender and blend everything well until a smooth dip forms.

3. Alternatively, you can Directions:the Ingredients: in a food processor as well.

4. Serve with your favorite fruit slices!

Nutrition Info:Per Serving: Calories: 148, Total Fat: 7.3 g, Saturated Fat: 1.8 g, Cholesterol: 1 mg, Sodium: 26 mg, Total Carbohydrate: 17 g, Dietary Fiber: 0.7 g, Total Sugars: 15 g, Protein: 5.9 g, Vitamin D: 0 mcg, Calcium: 37 mg, Iron: 0 mg, Potassium: 15 mg

Sun Dried Tomatoes, Dill And Feta Omelette Casserole

Servings: 6

Cooking Time: 40

Ingredients:

- 12 large eggs

- 2 cups whole milk

- 8 oz fresh spinach

- 2 cloves garlic, minced

- 12 oz artichoke salad with olives and peppers, drained and chopped

- 5 oz sun dried tomato feta cheese, crumbled

- 1 tbsp fresh chopped dill or 1 tsp dried dill

- 1 tsp dried oregano

- 1 tsp lemon pepper

- 1 tsp salt

- 4 tsp olive oil, divided

Directions:

1. Preheat oven to 375 degrees F

2. Chop the fresh herbs and artichoke salad

3. In a skillet over medium heat, add 1 tbsp olive oil

4. Sauté the spinach and garlic until wilted, about 3 minutes

5. Oil a 9x13 inch baking dish, layer the spinach and artichoke salad evenly in the dish

6. In a medium bowl, whisk together the eggs, milk, herbs, salt and lemon pepper

7. Pour the egg mixture over vegetables, sprinkle with feta cheese

8. Bake in the center of the oven for 35-40 minutes until firm in the center

9. Allow to cool, slice a and distribute among the storage containers. Store for 2-3 days or freeze for 3 months

10. To Serve: Reheat in the microwave for 30 seconds or until heated through or in the toaster oven for 5 minutes or until heated through

Nutrition Info:Per Serving: Calories:196;Total Carbohydrates: 5g;Total Fat: 12g;Protein: 10g

Lunch and Dinner Recipes

Roast Chicken

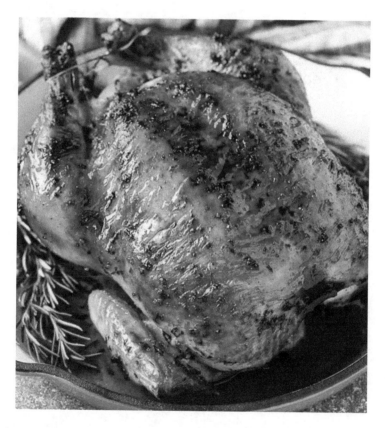

Servings: 6

Cooking Time: 1 – 1 ½ Hour

Ingredients:

- fresh orange juice, 1 large orange

- ¼ cup Dijon mustard

- ¼ cup olive oil

- 4 teaspoons dried Greek oregano

- salt

- ground black pepper

- 12 potatoes, peeled and cubed

- 5 garlic cloves, minced

- 1 whole chicken

Directions:

1. Preheat oven to 375 degrees F.

2. Take a bowl and whisk in orange juice, Greek oregano, Dijon mustard, salt, and pepper. Mix well.

3. Add potatoes to the bowl and coat them thoroughly.

4. Transfer the potatoes to a large baking dish, leaving remaining juice in a bowl.

5. Stuff the garlic cloves into your chicken (under the skin).

6. Place the chicken into the bowl with the remaining juice and coat it thoroughly.

7. Transfer chicken to the baking dish, placing it on top of the potatoes.

8. Pour any extra juice on top of chicken and potatoes.

9. Bake uncovered until the thickest part of the chicken registers 160 degrees F, and the juices run clear, anywhere from 60 – minutes.

10. Remove the chicken and cover it with doubled aluminum foil.

11. Allow it to rest for 10 minutes.

12. Slice, spread over containers and enjoy!

Nutrition Info:Per Serving: Calories: 1080, Total Fat: 36.4 g, Saturated Fat: 8.8 g, Cholesterol: 325 mg, Sodium: 458 mg, Total Carbohydrate: 70.5 g, Dietary Fiber: 11.1 g, Total Sugars: 6.3 g, Protein: 16 g, Vitamin D: 0 mcg, Calcium: 120 mg, Iron: 7 mg, Potassium: 2691 mg

Chicken Eggplant

Servings: 5

Cooking Time: 40 Minutes

Ingredients:

- 3 pieces of eggplants, peeled and cut up lengthwise into ½ inch slices

- 3 tablespoons olive oil

- 6 skinless and boneless chicken breast halves, diced

- 1 onion, diced

- 2 tablespoons tomato paste

- ½ cup water

- 2 teaspoons dried oregano

- salt

- pepper

Directions:

1. Place the eggplant strips in a large pot filled with lightly salted water.

2. Allow them to soak for 30 minutes.

3. Remove the eggplant from the pot and brush thoroughly with olive oil.

4. Heat a skillet over medium heat.

5. Add eggplant and sauté for a few minutes.

6. Transfer the sautéed eggplant to a baking dish.

7. Heat a large skillet over medium heat.

8. Add chicken, onion, and sauté.

9. Stir in water and tomato paste.

10. Reduce heat to low, cover, and simmer for minutes.

11. Preheat oven to 400 degrees F.

12. Pour the chicken tomato mix over your eggplant.

13. Season with oregano, pepper, and salt.

14. Cover with aluminum foil and bake for 20 minutes.

15. Cool, place to containers and chill.

Nutrition Info:Per Serving: Calories: 319, Total Fat: 11.3 g, Saturated Fat: 1.2 g, Cholesterol: 117 mg, Sodium: 143 mg, Total Carbohydrate: 7.2 g, Dietary Fiber: 3.1 g, Total Sugars: 3.5 g, Protein: 48 g, Vitamin D: 0 mcg, Calcium: 22 mg, Iron: 2 mg, Potassium: 244 mg

Grilled Steak

Servings: 2

Cooking Time: 15 Minutes

Ingredients:

- ¼ cup unsalted butter

- 2 garlic cloves, minced

- ¾ pound beef top sirloin steaks

- ¾ teaspoon dried rosemary, crushed

- 2 oz. parmesan cheese, shredded

- Salt and black pepper, to taste

Directions:

1. Preheat the grill and grease it.

2. Season the sirloin steaks with salt and black pepper.

3. Transfer the steaks on the grill and cook for about 5 minutes on each side.

4. Dish out the steaks in plates and keep aside.

5. Meanwhile, put butter and garlic in a pan and heat until melted.

6. Pour it on the steaks and serve hot.

7. Divide the steaks in 2 containers and refrigerate for about 3 days for meal prepping purpose. Reheat in microwave before serving.

Nutrition Info: Calories: 3 ;Carbohydrates: 1.5g ;Protein: 41.4g;Fat: 23.6g;Sugar: 0g;Sodium: 352mg

Beef And Veggie Lasagna

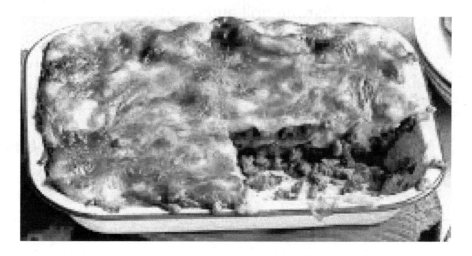

Servings: 10

Cooking Time: 1 Hour 10 Minutes

Ingredients:

- 3 teaspoons olive oil, divided

- 1 medium zucchini, quartered lengthwise and chopped (about 1⅓ cups)

- 3 cups packed baby spinach

- 1 cup chopped yellow onion

- 1 teaspoon chopped garlic

- 8 ounces button or cremini mushrooms, finely chopped

- 1 cup shredded carrots

- 8 ounces lean (90/10) ground beef

- ½ cup dry red wine

- 1 (28-ounce) can low-sodium or no-salt-added crushed tomatoes

- 1 (15-ounce) can tomato sauce

- ¼ teaspoon kosher salt

- 1 (16-ounce) container low-fat (2%) cottage cheese

- 1 large egg

- 3 tablespoons grated Parmesan cheese

- 2 cups shredded part-skim mozzarella cheese, divided

- ½ cup fresh basil leaves, chopped

- 1 (9-ounce) box oven-ready lasagna noodles

Directions:

1. Preheat the oven to 375°F.

2. Heat 1 teaspoon of oil in a 1inch skillet over medium-high heat. When the oil is shimmering, add the zucchini and cook for 2 minutes. Add the spinach and continue to cook for 1 more minute. Remove the veggies to a plate.

3. In the same skillet, heat the remaining 2 teaspoons of oil over medium-high heat. When the oil is hot, add the onion and garlic and cook for 2 minutes. Add the mushrooms and carrots and cook for 4 more minutes. Add the ground beef and continue cooking for 4 more minutes, until the meat has browned. Add the wine and cook for 1 minute. Add the crushed tomatoes,

tomato sauce, and salt, stir, and turn off the heat.

4. In a large mixing bowl, combine the cottage cheese, egg, and Parmesan, ½ cup of shredded cheese, and the basil.

5. Ladle 2 cups of sauce on the bottom of a 9-by-13-inch glass or ceramic baking dish. Place 4 noodles side by side in the pan. Layer 1 cup of sauce, half of the veggies, and half of the cottage cheese. Repeat with 4 more noodles, 1 cup of sauce, the remaining half of the veggies, and the remaining half of the cottage cheese. Top with 4 more noodles, the remainder of the sauce, and the remaining 1½ cups of shredded cheese.

6. Cover the pan with foil, trying not to touch the foil to the cheese, and bake for 40 minutes. Remove the foil and bake for 10 to 15 more minutes, until the cheese starts to brown.

7. When the lasagna cools, cut it into 10 pieces and place 1 piece in each of 10 containers.

8. STORAGE: Store covered containers in the refrigerator for up to 5 days. Cooked lasagna freezes well and can last for up to 3 months.

Nutrition Info:Per Serving: Total calories: 321; Total fat: 11g; Saturated fat: 4g; Sodium: 680mg; Carbohydrates: 34g; Fiber: 5g; Protein: 24g

Greek Shrimp And Farro Bowls

Servings: 4

Cooking Time: 20 Minutes

Ingredients:

- 1 lb peeled and deveined shrimp

- 3 Tbsp. extra virgin olive oil

- 2 cloves garlic, minced

- 2 bell peppers, sliced thick

- 2 medium-sized zucchinis, sliced into thin rounds

- pint cherry tomatoes, halved

- ¼ cup thinly sliced green or black olives

- 4 Tbsp. 2% reduced-fat plain Greek yogurt

- Juice of 1 lemon

- 2 tsp fresh chopped dill

- 1 Tbsp. fresh chopped oregano

- ½ tsp smoked paprika

- ½ tsp sea salt

- ¼ tsp black pepper

- 1 cup dry farro

Directions:

1. In a bowl, add the olive oil, garlic, lemon, dill, oregano, paprika, salt, and pepper, whisk to combine

2. Pour 3/4 the amount of marinade over shrimp, toss to coat and all to stand 10 minutes

3. Reserve the rest of the marinade for later

4. Cook the farro according to package instructions in water or chicken stock

5. In a grill pan or nonstick skillet over medium heat, add the olive

6. Once heated, add shrimp, cook for 2-3 minutes per side, until no longer pink, then transfer to a plate

7. Working in batches, cook bell pepper, zucchinis, and cherry tomatoes to the grill pan or skillet, cook for 5-6 minutes, until softened

8. allow the dish to cool completely

9. Distribute the farro among the containers, evenly add the shrimp, grilled vegetables, olives, and tomatoes, store for 2 days

10. To Serve: Reheat in the microwave for 1-2 minutes or until heated through. Drizzle the reserved marinade over top. Top each bowl with 1 tbsp Greek yogurt and extra lemon juice, if desired

Nutrition Info:Per Serving: Calories:428;Carbs: 45g;Total Fat: 13g;Protein: 34g

Asparagus Salmon Fillets

Servings: 2

Cooking Time: 30 Minutes

Ingredients:

- 1 teaspoon olive oil

- 4 asparagus stalks

- 2 salmon fillets

- ¼ cup butter

- ¼ cup champagne

- Salt and freshly ground black pepper, to taste

Directions:

1. Preheat the oven to 355 degrees F and grease a baking dish.

2. Put all the ingredients in a bowl and mix well.

3. Put this mixture in the baking dish and transfer it in the oven.

4. Bake for about 20 minutes and dish out.

5. Place the salmon fillets in a dish and keep aside to cool for meal prepping. Divide it into 2 containers and close the lid. Refrigerate for 1 day and reheat in microwave before serving.

Nutrition Info: Calories: 475 ;Carbohydrates: 1.1g;Protein: 35.2g;Fat: 38g;Sugar: 0.5g;Sodium: 242mg

Grilled Calamari With Berries

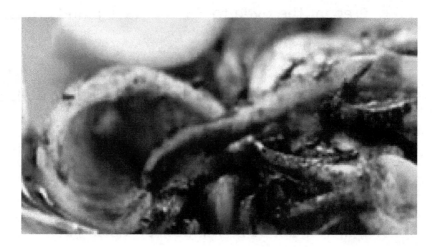

Servings: 4

Cooking Time: 5 Minutes

Ingredients:

- ¼ cup olive oil

- ¼ cup extra virgin olive oil

- 1 thinly sliced apple

- ¾ cup blueberries

- ¼ cup sliced almonds

- 1 ½ pounds calamari tube

- ¼ cup dried cranberries

- 6 cups spinach

- 2 tablespoons apple cider vinegar

- 1 tablespoon lemon juice

- Sea salt and pepper to your liking

Directions:

1. Start by making the vinaigrette. Combine apple cider vinegar, lemon juice, extra virgin olive oil, sea salt, and pepper. Whisk well and set aside.

2. Set your grill to medium heat.

3. In a separate bowl, add the calamari tube and mix with salt, pepper, and olive oil.

4. Set the calamari on the grill and cook both sides for 2 to 3 minutes.

5. In another bowl, mix the salad by adding the spinach, cranberries, almonds, blueberries, and apples. Toss to mix.

6. Set the cooked calamari onto a cutting board and let it cool for a few minutes. Cut them into ¼-inch thick rings and then toss them into the salad bowl.

7. Sprinkle the vinaigrette sauce onto the salad. Toss to mix the ingredients and enjoy!

Nutrition Info: calories: 567, fats: 24.4 grams, carbohydrates: 30 grams, protein: 55 grams.

Italian Sausage And Veggie Pizza Pasta

Servings: 8

Cooking Time: 30 Minutes

Ingredients:

- 1 tsp olive oil

- 1 (2.25 oz) can of sliced black olives

- 1 (28 oz) can of tomato sauce

- 1 (16 oz) box penne pasta

- 3 cups water

- 3 sweet Italian sausage links, casings removed, around 1 lb of sausage

- 1 cup sliced onions

- 1 cup sliced green bell pepper

- 2-3 garlic cloves, minced or pressed

- 8 oz. sliced mushrooms

- 1/2 cup Pepperoni, cut in half and then each half cut into thirds + a few extra whole pieces for topping

- 1/2 tsp Italian seasoning

- 1/2 tsp salt

- Salt, to taste

- Pepper to taste

- 2 cups shredded mozzarella cheese, divided

- Garnish:

- Chopped fresh parsley and Romano cheese

Directions:

1. In a deep heavy-bottom, oven-safe pot over medium heat, add the oil

2. Once heated, add in the sausage and break it up with a wooden spoon

3. Then add in the onions, peppers, garlic and mushrooms, stir to combine, season with salt and pepper to taste. Sauté until the sausage crumbles have browned, stirring frequently for around 10 minutes

4. Add in the pepperoni and olives to the pan, sauté for 1-2 minutes.

5. Then add in the sauce, water, Italian seasoning, salt and pasta to the pan, stir to combine

6. Bring the pot to a boil

7. Once boiling, reduce the heat to medium low, cover and allow to simmer for 10 minutes, stirring occasionally

8. Remove the cover and continue to simmer for 3-5 minutes, stirring occasionally

9. Stir in 1/2 cup of shredded Mozzarella cheese, sprinkle the remaining cheese on top

10. Arrange a few more whole pepperonis on top of the cheese, broil for a few minutes until the cheese is bubbling and melted

11. Top with the parsley and Romano cheese

12. Allow to cool and distribute the pasta evenly among the containers. Store in the fridge for 3-4 days or in the freezer for 2 weeks.

13. To Serve: Reheat in the oven at 375 degrees for 1-2 minutes or until heated through.

14. Recipe Note: If you would like it to be spicy, you can also use hot Italian sausage.

Nutrition Info:Per Serving: Calories:450;Total Fat: 21.9g;Total Carbs: 22g;Fiber: 5g;Protein: 43g

Baked Chicken Thighs With Lemon, Olives, And Brussels Sprouts

Servings: 4

Cooking Time: 40 Minutes

Ingredients:

- 2 tablespoons olive oil, divided

- 1 pound Brussels sprouts, stemmed and halved (quartered if the sprouts are extra large)

- 1 pound boneless, skinless chicken thighs

- 2 teaspoons chopped garlic

- 1 teaspoon dried oregano

- ½ teaspoon kosher salt

- 3 tablespoons freshly squeezed lemon juice

- ½ cup pitted kalamata olives

Directions:

1. Preheat the oven to 350°F.

2. Spread 1 tablespoon of oil over the bottom of a 13-by-9-inch glass or ceramic baking dish. Add the Brussels sprouts to the pan and spread out evenly. Place the chicken on top of the sprouts and rub the garlic and oregano into the top of the chicken.

3. Sprinkle the salt, the remaining 1 tablespoon of oil, the lemon juice, and the olives over the contents of the pan.

4. Cover the pan with aluminum foil and bake for 20 minutes. Remove the foil and bake uncovered for 20 more minutes. Cool.

5. Place one quarter of the chicken and ¾ cup of Brussels sprouts in each of 4 containers. Drizzle any remaining juices from the pan over the chicken.

6. STORAGE: Store covered containers in the refrigerator for 5 days.

Nutrition Info:Per Serving: Total calories: 28 Total fat: 18g; Saturated fat: 3g; Sodium: 737mg; Carbohydrates: 14g; Fiber: 5g; Protein: 20g

Slow Cooker Lamb, Herb, And Bean Stew

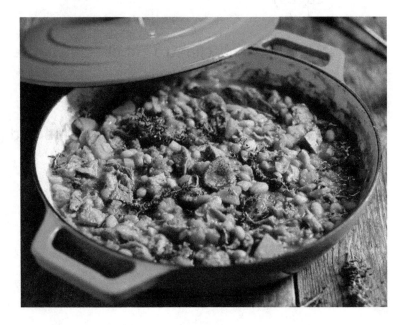

Servings: 4

Cooking Time: 15 Minutes

Ingredients:

- 3 bunches of parsley (about 6 packed cups of leaves)

- 1 large bunch cilantro (about 1½ packed cups of leaves)

- 1 bunch scallions, sliced (both white and green parts, about 1¼ cups)

- 1 pound leg of lamb, fat trimmed, cut into 1-inch pieces

- 2 tablespoons olive oil, divided

- 1 medium onion, chopped

- 2 teaspoons chopped garlic

- 2 teaspoons turmeric

- ¾ teaspoon kosher salt

- 2 tablespoons tomato paste

- 2½ cups low-sodium chicken broth

- 2 (15.5-ounce) cans low-sodium kidney beans, drained and rinsed

- 2 tablespoons freshly squeezed lemon juice

Directions:

1. Finely chop the parsley leaves, cilantro leaves, and scallions with a knife, or pulse in the food processor until finely chopped but not puréed. With this amount of herbs, you'll need to pulse in two batches.

2. Pat the lamb cubes with a paper towel. Heat a 1inch skillet over medium-high heat and add 1 tablespoon of oil. Once the oil is shimmering, add the lamb and brown for 5 minutes, flipping after 3 minutes. Place the lamb in the slow cooker.

3. Turn the heat down to medium and add the remaining 1 tablespoon of oil to the skillet. Once the oil is hot, add the onions and garlic

and sauté for minutes. Add the turmeric, salt, and tomato paste and continue to cook for 2 more minutes, stirring frequently.

4. Add the chopped parsley, cilantro, and scallions. Sauté for 5 minutes, stirring occasionally.

5. While the herbs are cooking, add the broth, beans, and lemon juice to the slow cooker. Add the herb mixture when it's done cooking on the stove. Turn the slow cooker to the low setting and cook for 8 hours.

6. Taste and add more salt and/or lemon juice if needed. Cool.

7. Scoop 2 cups of stew into each of 4 containers.

8. STORAGE: Store covered containers in the refrigerator for up to 5 days. Stew can be frozen for up to 4 months.

Nutrition Info:Per Serving: Total calories: 486; Total fat: 15g; Saturated fat: 5g; Sodium: 6mg; Carbohydrates: 51g; Fiber: 15g; Protein: 41g

Holiday Chicken Salad

Servings: 2

Cooking Time: 25 Minutes

Ingredients:

- 1 celery stalk, chopped

- 1½ cups cooked grass-fed chicken, chopped

- ¼ cup fresh cranberries

- ¼ cup sour cream

- ½ apple, chopped

- ¼ yellow onion, chopped

- 1/8 cup almonds, toasted and chopped

- 2-ounce feta cheese, crumbled

- ¼ cup avocado mayonnaise

- Salt and black pepper, to taste

Directions:

1. Stir together all the ingredients in a bowl except almonds and cheese.

2. Top with almonds and cheese to serve.

3. Meal Prep Tip: Don't add almonds and cheese in the salad if you want to store the salad. Cover with a plastic wrap and refrigerate to serve.

Nutrition Info: Calories: 336 ;Carbohydrates: 8.8g;Protein: 25g;Fat: 23.2g ;Sugar: 5.4g;Sodium: 383mg

Costa Brava Chicken

Servings: 4

Cooking Time: 35 Minutes

Ingredients:

- 1 20-ounce can pineapple chunks

- 10 skinless and boneless chicken breast halves

- 1 tablespoon vegetable oil

- 1 teaspoon ground cumin

- 1 teaspoon ground cinnamon

- 2garlic cloves, minced

- 1 onion, quartered

- 1 14-ounce can stewed tomatoes

- 2 cups black olives

- ½ cup salsa

- 2 tablespoons water

- 1 red bell pepper, thinly sliced

- salt

Directions:

1. Drain the pineapple chunks, but be sure to reserve the juice.

2. Sprinkle pineapples with salt.

3. Heat oil in a large frying pan over medium heat.

4. Add the chicken and cook until brown.

5. Combine the cinnamon and cumin and sprinkle over the chicken.

6. Add garlic and onion and cook until the onions are tender.

7. Add reserved pineapple juices, olives, tomatoes, and salsa.

8. Reduce heat, cover, and allow to simmer for 25 minutes.

9. Combine the cornstarch and water in a bowl.

10. Add the cornstarch mixture to the pan and stir.

11. Add the bell pepper and simmer for a little longer until the sauce bubbles and thickens.

12. Stir in pineapple chunks until thoroughly heated.

13. Enjoy!

Nutrition Info:Per Serving: Calories: 651, Total Fat: 16.5 g, Saturated Fat: 1.7 g, Cholesterol: 228 mg, Sodium: 1053 mg, Total Carbohydrate: 34.7 g, Dietary Fiber: 7.2 g, Total Sugars: 20.3 g, Protein: 94.5 g, Vitamin D: 0 mcg, Calcium: 118 mg, Iron: 6 mg, Potassium: 606 mg

One Skillet Greek Lemon Chicken And Rice

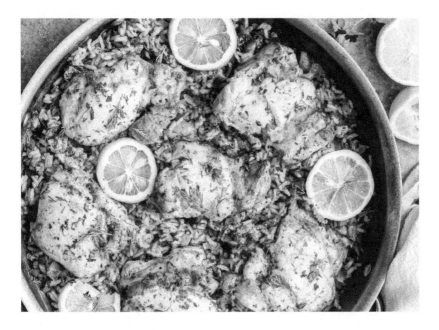

Servings: 5

Cooking Time: 45 Minutes

Ingredients:

- Marinade:

- 2 tsp dried oregano

- 1 tsp dried minced onion

- 4-5 cloves garlic, minced

- Zest of 1 lemon

- 1/2 tsp kosher salt

- 1/2 tsp black pepper

- 1-2 Tbsp olive oil to make a loose paste

- 5 bone-in, skin on chicken thighs

- Rice:

- 1 1/2 Tbsp olive oil

- 1 large yellow onion, peeled and diced

- 1 cup dry long-grain white rice (NOT minute or quick cooking varieties)

- 2 cups chicken stock

- 1 1/4 tsp dried oregano

- 5 cloves garlic, minced

- 3/4 tsp kosher salt

- 1/2 tsp black pepper

- Lemon slices, optional

- Fresh minced parsley, for garnish

- Extra lemon zest, for garnish

Directions:

1. In a large resealable plastic bag, add the oregano, dried minced onion, garlic, lemon zest, salt, black pepper, and olive oil, massage to combine

2. Add chicken thighs, and then turn/massage to coat, refrigerate 15 minutes or overnight

3. Preheat oven to 0 F degrees

4. In a large cast iron or heavy oven safe skillet over medium-high heat, add 1 1/2 Tbsp olive oil to

5. Remove the chicken thighs from the refrigerator, shake off the excess marinade and add chicken thighs, skin side down, to pan, cook 4-minutes per side

6. Transfer to a plate and wipe the skillet lightly with a paper towel to remove any burnt bits, reserving chicken grease in pan.

7. Lower the heat to medium and add onion to pan, cook 3-4 minutes, until softened and slightly charred. Add in garlic and cook 1 minute

8. Then add in the rice, oregano, salt and pepper, stir together and cook for 1 minute

9. Pour in chicken stock, turn the temperature up to medium-high, bring to a simmer

10. Once simmering, place the chicken thighs on top of the rice mixture, push down gently

11. Cover with lid or foil, and bake 35 minutes

12. Uncover, return to oven and bake an additional 10-15 minutes, until liquid is removed, the rice is tender, and chicken is cooked through

13. Allow the rice and chicken to cool

14. Distribute among the containers, store in fridge for 2-3 days

15. To serve: Reheat in the microwave for 1 minute to 2 minutes or cooked through. Garnish with lemon zest and parsley, and serve!

Nutrition Info:Per Serving: Calories:325;Carbs: 35g;Total Fat: 11g;Protein: 21g

Trout With Wilted Greens

Servings: 4

Cooking Time: 15 Minutes

Ingredients:

- 2 teaspoons extra virgin olive oil

- 2 cups kale, chopped

- 2 cups Swiss chard, chopped

- ½ sweet onion, thinly sliced

- 4 (5 ounce boneless skin-on trout fillets)

- Juice of 1 lemon

- Sea salt

- Freshly ground pepper

- Zest of 1 lemon

Directions:

1. Pre-heat your oven to 375-degree Fahrenheit

2. Lightly grease a 9 by 13-inch baking dish with olive oil

3. Arrange the kale, Swiss chard, onion in a dish

4. Top greens with fish, skin side up and drizzle with olive oil and lemon juice

5. Season fish with salt and pepper

6. Bake for 15 minutes until fish flakes

7. Sprinkle zest

8. Serve and enjoy!

9. Meal Prep/Storage Options: Store in airtight containers in your fridge for 1-3 days.

Nutrition Info: Calories: 315;Fat: 14g;Carbohydrates: 6g;Protein: 39g

One Skillet Chicken In Roasted Red Pepper Sauce

Servings: 4

Cooking Time: 20 Minutes

Ingredients:

- 4-6 boneless skinless chicken thighs or breasts

- 2/3 cup chopped roasted red peppers (see note)

- 2 tsp Italian seasoning, divided

- 4 tbsp oil

- 1 tbsp minced garlic

- 1/2 tsp salt

- 1/4 tsp black pepper

- 1 cup heavy cream

- 2 tbsp crumbled feta cheese, optional

- Thinly sliced fresh basil, optional

Directions:

1. In a blender or food processer, combine the roasted red peppers, tsp Italian seasoning, oil, garlic, salt, and pepper, pulse until smooth.

2. In a large skillet over medium heat, add the olive oil and season chicken with remaining 1 tsp Italian seasoning. Cook chicken for 6-8 minutes on each side, or until cooked through and lightly browned on the outside. Then transfer to a plate and cover

3. Add the red pepper mixture to the pan, stir over medium heat 2-minutes, or until heated throughout. Add the heavy cream, stir until mixture is thick and creamy

4. Add chicken, toss in the sauce to coat

5. allow the dish to cool completely

6. Distribute among the containers, store for 2-3 days

7. To Serve: Reheat in the microwave for 1-2 minutes or until heated through. Garnish with crumbled feta cheese and fresh basil. Serve with your favorite grain.

8. Recipe Notes: You can purchase jarred roasted red peppers at most grocery stores around the olives.

Nutrition Info:Per Serving: Calories:655;Carbs: 12g;Total Fat: 25g;Protein: 8

Mediterranean Minestrone Soup

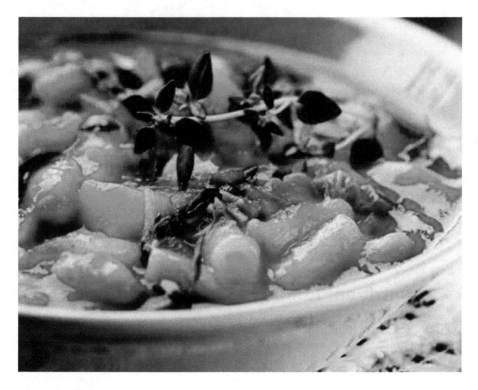

Servings: 4

Cooking Time: 40 Minutes

Ingredients:

- 1 large onion, finely chopped

- 4 cups vegetable stock

- 4 cloves crushed garlic

- 1 ounce chopped carrots

- 4 ounces chopped red bell pepper

- 4 ounces chopped celery (keep leaves)

- 1 16-ounce can diced tomatoes

- 1 16-ounce can white beans

- 4 ounces fresh spinach, chopped

- 4 ounces multi-colored pasta

- 2 ounces grated parmesan

  - 2 tablespoons olive oil

- bunch of chopped parsley

- 1 teaspoon dried oregano

- salt

- pepper

- 4 ounces salami, finely sliced (if desired)

Directions:

1. Heat oil in a pan over medium heat.

2. Add chopped onions, red pepper, carrots, and celery.

3. Saute for about 10 minutes until tender.

4. Add garlic and cook on low heat for 2 minutes more.

5. Add your stock and tomatoes and cook for an additional 10 minutes.

6. Add pasta and cook for 15 minutes more until al dente.

7. Taste / check your seasoning; add salt and pepper as needed.

8. Add parsley, beans, celery leaves, spinach, and salami (if using), and stir.

9. Pour the whole mixture to a boil and stir for about 2 minutes.

10. Enjoy the soup hot!

Nutrition Info:Per Serving: Calories: 888, Total Fat: 19.9 g, Saturated Fat: 6.3 g, Cholesterol: 30 mg, Sodium: 1200 mg, Total Carbohydrate: 139.5 g, Dietary Fiber: 31.8 g, Total Sugars: 14.3 g, Protein: 49.4 g, Vitamin D: 14 mcg, Calcium: 64.3 mg, Iron: 22 mg, Potassium: 3951 mg

Baked Shrimp Stew

Servings: 4-6

Cooking Time: 25 Minutes

Ingredients:

- Greek extra virgin olive oil

- 2 1/2 lb prawns, peeled, deveined, rinsed well and dried

- 1 large red onion, chopped (about two cups)

- 5 garlic cloves, roughly chopped

- 1 red bell pepper, seeded, chopped

- 2 15-oz cans diced tomatoes

- 1/2 cup water

- 1 1/2 tsp ground coriander

- 1 tsp sumac

- 1 tsp cumin

- 1 tsp red pepper flakes, more to taste

- 1/2 tsp ground green cardamom

- Salt and pepper, to taste

- 1 cup parsley leaves, stems removed

- 1/3 cup toasted pine nuts

- 1/4 cup toasted sesame seeds

- Lemon or lime wedges to serve

Directions:

1. Preheat the oven to 375 degrees F

2. In a large frying pan, add 1 tbsp olive oil

3. Sauté the prawns for 2 minutes, until they are barely pink, then remove and set aside

4. In the same pan over medium-high heat, drizzle a little more olive oil and sauté the chopped onions, garlic and red bell peppers for 5 minutes, stirring regularly

5. Add in the canned diced tomatoes and water, allow to simmer for 10 minutes, until the liquid reduces, stir occasionally

6. Reduce the heat to medium, add the shrimp back to the pan, stir in the spices the ground coriander, sumac, cumin, red pepper flakes, green cardamom, salt and pepper, then the toasted pine nuts, sesame seeds and parsley leaves, stir to combined

7. Transfer the shrimp and sauce to an oven-safe earthenware or stoneware dish, cover tightly with foil Place in the oven to bake for minutes, uncover and broil briefly.

8. allow the dish to cool completely

9. Distribute among the containers, store for 2-3 days

10. To Serve: Reheat on the stove for 1-2 minutes or until heated through. Serve with your favorite bread or whole grain. Garnish with a side of lime or lemon wedges.

Nutrition Info:Per Serving: Calories:377;Carbs: ;Total Fat: 20g;Protein: 41g

Rainbow Salad With Roasted Chickpeas

Servings: 2-3

Cooking Time: 40 Minutes

Ingredients:

- Creamy avocado dressing, store bought or homemade

- 3 large tri-color carrots - one orange, one red, and one yellow

- 1 medium zucchini

- 1/4 cup fresh basil, cut into ribbons

- 1 can chickpeas, rinsed and drained

- 1 tbsp olive oil

- 1 tsp chili powder

- 1/2 tsp cumin

- Salt, to taste

- Pepper, to taste

Directions:

1. Preheat the oven to 400 degrees F

2. Pat the chickpeas dry with paper towels

3. Add them to a bowl and toss with the olive oil, chili powder, cumin, and salt and pepper

4. Arrange the chickpeas on a baking sheet in a single layer

5. Bake for 30-40 minutes - making sure to shaking the pan once in a while to prevent over browning. The chickpeas will be done when they're crispy and golden brown, allow to cool

6. With a grater, peeler, mandolin or spiralizer, shred the carrots and zucchini into very thin ribbons

7. Once the zucchini is shredded, lightly press it with paper towels to remove excess moisture

8. Add the shredded zucchini and carrots to a bowl, toss with the basil

9. Add in the roasted chickpeas, too gently to combine

10. Distribute among the containers, store for 2 days

11. To Serve: Top with the avocado dressing and enjoy

Nutrition Info:Per Serving: (without dressing): Calories:640;Total Fat: 51g;Total Carbs: 9.8g;Protein: 38.8g

Sour And Sweet Fish

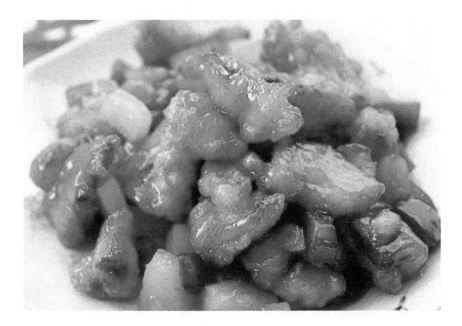

Servings: 2

Cooking Time: 25 Minutes

Ingredients:

- 1 tablespoon vinegar

- 2 drops stevia

- 1 pound fish chunks

- ¼ cup butter, melted

- Salt and black pepper, to taste

Directions:

1. Put butter and fish chunks in a skillet and cook for about 3 minutes.

2. Add stevia, salt and black pepper and cook for about 10 minutes, stirring continuously.

3. Dish out in a bowl and serve immediately.

4. Place fish in a dish and set aside to cool for meal prepping. Divide it in 2 containers and refrigerate for up to 2 days. Reheat in microwave before serving.

Nutrition Info: Calories: 2 ;Carbohydrates: 2.8g;Protein: 24.5g;Fat: 16.7g;Sugar: 2.7g;Sodium: 649mg

Papaya Mangetout Stew

Servings: 2

Cooking Time: 5 Minutes

Ingredients:

- 2 cups Mangetout

- 2 cups bean sprouts

- 1 tablespoon water

- 1 papaya, peeled, deseeded, and cubed

- 1 lime, juiced

- 2 tablespoon unsalted peanuts

- small handful basil leaves, torn

- small handful mint leaves, chopped

Directions:

1. Take a large frying pan and place it over high heat.

2. Add Mangetout, 1 tablespoon of water, and bean sprouts.

3. Cook for about 2-minutes.

4. Remove from heat, add papaya, and lime juice.

5. Toss everything well.

6. Spread over containers.

7. Before eating, garnish with herbs and peanuts.

8. Enjoy!

Nutrition Info:Per Serving: Calories: 283, Total Fat: 6.4 g, Saturated Fat: 0.g, Cholesterol: 0 mg, Sodium: 148 mg, Total Carbohydrate: 42.8 g, Dietary Fiber: 4.9 g, Total Sugars: 21.5 g, Protein: 20.1 g, Vitamin D: 0 mcg, Calcium: 205 mg, Iron: 3 mg, Potassium: 743 mg

Mediterranean Pork Pita Sandwich

Servings: 6

Cooking Time: 10 Minutes

Ingredients:

- 2 teaspoons olive oil, plus 1 tablespoon

- 2 cups packed baby spinach leaves, finely chopped

- 4 ounces mushrooms, finely chopped

- 1 teaspoon chopped garlic

- 1 pound extra-lean ground pork

- 1 large egg

- ½ cup panko bread crumbs

- ⅓ cup chopped fresh dill

97

- ¼ teaspoon kosher salt

- 6 large romaine lettuce leaves, ripped into pieces to fit pita

- 2 tomatoes, sliced

- 3 whole-wheat pitas, cut in half

- ¾ cup Garlic Yogurt Sauce

Directions:

1. Heat 2 teaspoons of oil in a -inch skillet over medium heat. Once the oil is shimmering, add the spinach, mushrooms, and garlic and sauté for 3 minutes. Cool for 5 minutes.

2. Place the mushroom mixture in a large mixing bowl and add the pork, egg, bread crumbs, dill, and salt. Mix with your hands until everything is well combined. Make 6 patties, about ½-inch thick and 3 inches in diameter.

3. Heat the remaining 1 tablespoon of oil in the same 12-inch skillet over medium-high heat. When the oil is hot, add the patties. They should all be able to fit in the pan. If not, cook in 2 batches. Cook for 5 minutes on the first side and 4 minutes on the second side. The outside should be golden brown, and the inside should no longer be pink.

4. Place 1 patty in each of 6 containers. In each of 6 separate containers that will not be reheated, place 1 torn lettuce leaf and 2 tomato slices. Wrap the pita halves in plastic wrap and place one in each veggie container. Spoon 2 tablespoons of yogurt sauce into each of 6 sauce containers.

5. STORAGE: Store covered containers in the refrigerator for up to days. Uncooked patties can be frozen for up to 4 months, while cooked patties can be frozen for up to 3 months.

Nutrition Info:Per Serving: Total calories: 309; Total fat: 11g; Saturated fat: 3g; Sodium: 343mg; Carbohydrates: 22g; Fiber: 3g; Protein: 32g

Salmon With Warm Tomato-olive Salad

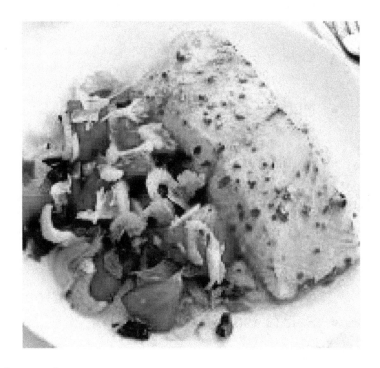

Servings: 4

Cooking Time: 25 Minutes

Ingredients:

- Salmon fillets (4/approx. 4 oz./1.25-inches thick)

- Celery (1 cup)

- Medium tomatoes (2)

- Fresh mint (.25 cup)

- Kalamata olives (.5 cup)

- Garlic (.5 tsp.)

- Salt (1 tsp. + more to taste)

- Honey (1 tbsp.)

- Red pepper flakes (.25 tsp.)

- Olive oil (2 tbsp. + more for the pan)

- Vinegar (1 tsp.)

Directions:

1. Slice the tomatoes and celery into inch pieces and mince the garlic. Chop the mint and the olives.

2. Heat the oven using the broiler setting.

3. Whisk the oil, vinegar, honey, red pepper flakes, and salt (1 tsp.. Brush the mixture onto the salmon.

4. Line the broiler pan with a sheet of foil. Spritz the pan lightly with olive oil, and add the fillets (skin side downward.

5. Broil them for four to six minutes until well done.

6. Meanwhile, make the tomato salad. Mix ½ teaspoon of the salt with the garlic.

7. Prepare a small saucepan on the stovetop using the med-high temperature setting. Pour in the rest of the oil and add the garlic mixture with

the olives and one tablespoon of vinegar. Simmer for about three minutes.

8. Prepare the serving dishes. Pour the bubbly mixture into the bowl and add the mint, tomato, and celery. Dust it with the salt as desired and toss.

9. When the salmon is done, serve with a tomato salad.

Nutrition Info: Calories: 433;Protein: 38 grams;Fat: 26 grams

Sauces and Dressings Recipes

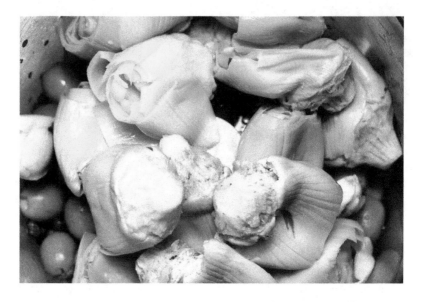

Servings: 1⅓ Cups

Cooking Time: 15 Minutes

Ingredients:

- 1 (6-ounce) jar marinated artichoke hearts, chopped

- ⅓ cup chopped pitted green olives (8 to 9 olives)

- 3 tablespoons chopped fresh basil

- ½ teaspoon freshly squeezed lemon juice

- 2 teaspoons olive oil

Directions:

1. Place all the ingredients in a medium mixing bowl and stir to combine.

2. Place the compote in a container and refrigerate.

3. STORAGE: Store the covered container in the refrigerator for up to 7 days.

4. Nutrition Info:Per Serving (⅓ cup): Total calories: 8 Total fat: 7g; Saturated fat: 1g; Sodium: 350mg; Carbohydrates: 5g; Fiber: <1g; Protein: <1g

Soups and Salads Recipes

Creamy Cilantro Lime Coleslaw

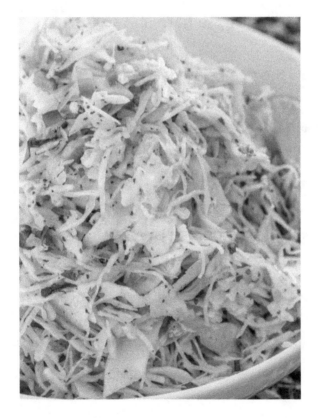

Servings: 2

Cooking Time: 10 Minutes

Ingredients:

- ¾ avocado

- 1 lime, juiced

- 1/8 cup water

- Cilantro, to garnish

- 6 oz coleslaw, bagged

- 1/8 cup cilantro leaves

- 1 garlic clove

- ¼ teaspoon salt

Directions:

1. Put garlic and cilantro in a food processor and process until chopped.

2. Add lime juice, avocado and water and pulse until creamy.

3. Put coleslaw in a large bowl and stir in the avocado mixture.

4. Refrigerate for a few hours before serving.

Nutrition Info: Calories: 240;Carbs: 17.4g;Fats: 19.6g;Proteins: 2.8g;Sodium: 0mg;Sugar: 0.5g

Snap Pea Salad

Servings: 2

Cooking Time: 15 Minutes

Ingredients:

- 1/8 cup lemon juice

- ½ clove garlic, crushed

- 4 ounces cauliflower riced

- 1/8 cup olive oil

- ¼ teaspoon coarse grain Dijon mustard

- ½ teaspoon granulated stevia

- ¼ cup sugar snap peas, ends removed and each pod cut into three pieces

- 1/8 cup chives

- 1/8 cup red onions, minced

- Sea salt and black pepper, to taste

- ¼ cup almonds, sliced

Directions:

1. Pour water in a pot fitted with a steamer basket and bring water to a boil.

2. Place riced cauliflower in the steamer basket and season with sea salt.

3. Cover the pot and steam for about 10 minutes until tender.

4. Drain the cauliflower and dish out in a bowl to refrigerate for about 1 hour.

5. Meanwhile, make a dressing by mixing olive oil, lemon juice, garlic, mustard, stevia, salt and black pepper in a bowl.

6. Mix together chilled cauliflower, peas, chives, almonds and red onions in another bowl.

7. Pour the dressing over this mixture and serve.

Nutrition Info: Calories: 203;Carbs: 7.6g;Fats: 18g;Proteins: 4.2g;Sodium: 28mg;Sugar: 2.9g

Spinach And Bacon Salad

Servings: 4

Cooking Time: 15 Minutes

Ingredients:

- 2 eggs, boiled, halved, and sliced

- 10 oz. organic baby spinach, rinsed, and dried

- 8 pieces thick bacon, cooked and sliced

- ½ cup plain mayonnaise

- ½ medium red onion, thinly sliced

Directions:

1. Mix together the mayonnaise and spinach in a large bowl.

2. Stir in the rest of the ingredients and combine well.

3. Dish out in a glass bowl and serve well.

Nutrition Info: Calories: 373;Carbs: ;Fats: 34.5g;Proteins: 11g;Sodium: 707mg;Sugar: 1.1g

Desserts Recipes

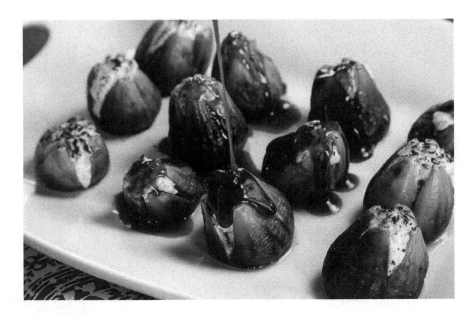

Servings: 6

Cooking Time: 20 Minutes

Ingredients:

- 10 halved fresh figs

- 20 chopped almonds

- 4 ounces goat cheese, divided

- 2 tablespoons of raw honey

Directions:

1. Turn your oven to broiler mode and set it to a high temperature.

2. Place your figs, cut side up, on a baking sheet. If you like to place a piece of parchment paper on top you can do this, but it is not necessary.

3. Sprinkle each fig with half of the goat cheese.

4. Add a tablespoon of chopped almonds to each fig.

5. Broil the figs for 3 to 4 minutes.

6. Take them out of the oven and let them cool for 5 to 7 minutes.

7. Sprinkle with the remaining goat cheese and honey.

Nutrition Info: calories: 209, fats: 9 grams, carbohydrates: 26 grams, protein: grams.

Chia Pudding With Strawberries

Servings: 4

Cooking Time: 4 Hours 5 Minutes

Ingredients:

- 2 cups unsweetened almond milk

- 1 tablespoon vanilla extract

- 2 tablespoons raw honey

- ¼ cup chia seeds

- 2 cups fresh and sliced strawberries

Directions:

1. In a medium bowl, combine the honey, chia seeds, vanilla, and unsweetened almond milk. Mix well.

2. Set the mixture in the refrigerator for at least 4 hours.

3. When you serve the pudding, top it with strawberries. You can even create a design in a glass serving bowl or dessert dish by adding a little pudding on the bottom, a few strawberries, top the strawberries with some more pudding, and then top the dish with a few strawberries.

Nutrition Info: calories: 108, fats: grams, carbohydrates: 17 grams, protein: 3 grams.

Meat Recipes

Grilled Chicken Salad With Avocado

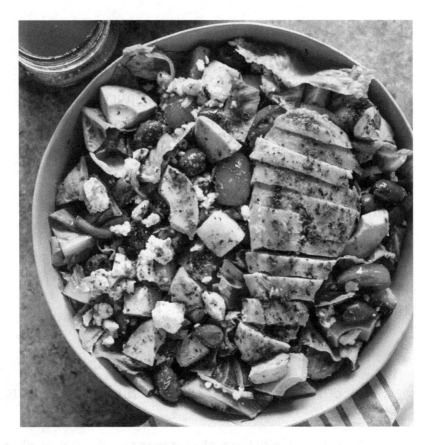

Servings: 4

Cooking Time: 20 Minutes

Ingredients:

- 1/3 cup olive oil

- 2 chicken breasts

- Sea salt and crushed red pepper flakes

- 2 egg yolks

- 1 tablespoon fresh lemon juice

- 1/2 teaspoon celery seeds

- 1 tablespoon coconut aminos

- 1 large-sized avocado, pitted and sliced

Directions:

1. Grill the chicken breasts for about 4 minutes per side. Season with salt and pepper, to taste.

2. Slice the grilled chicken into bite-sized strips.

3. To make the dressing, whisk the egg yolks, lemon juice, celery seeds, olive oil and coconut aminos in a measuring cup.

4. Storing

5. Place the chicken breasts in airtight containers or Ziploc bags; keep in your refrigerator for 3 to 4 days.

6. For freezing, place the chicken breasts in airtight containers or heavy-duty freezer bags. It will maintain the best quality for about 4 months. Defrost in the refrigerator.

7. Store dressing in your refrigerator for 3 to 4 days. Dress the salad and garnish with fresh avocado. Bon appétit!

Nutrition Info: 40Calories; 34.2g Fat; 4.8g Carbs; 22.7g Protein; 3.1g Fiber

Easy Fall-off-the-bone Ribs

Servings: 4

Cooking Time: 8 Hours

Ingredients:

- 1 pound baby back ribs

- 4 tablespoons coconut aminos

- 1/4 cup dry red wine

- 1/2 teaspoon cayenne pepper

- 1 garlic clove, crushed

- 1 teaspoon Italian herb mix

- 1 tablespoon butter

- 1 teaspoon Serrano pepper, minced

- 1 Italian pepper, thinly sliced

- 1 teaspoon grated lemon zest

Directions:

1. Butter the sides and bottom of your Crock pot. Place the pork and peppers on the bottom.

2. Add in the remaining ingredients.

3. Slow cook for 9 hours on Low heat setting.

4. Storing

5. Divide the baby back ribs into four portions. Place each portion of the ribs along with the peppers in an airtight container; keep in your refrigerator for 3 to days.

6. For freezing, place the ribs in airtight containers or heavy-duty freezer bags. Freeze up to 4 to months. Defrost in the refrigerator. Reheat in your oven at 250 degrees F until heated through.

Nutrition Info: 192 Calories; 6.9g Fat; 0.9g Carbs; 29.8g Protein; 0.5g Fiber

Brie-stuffed Meatballs

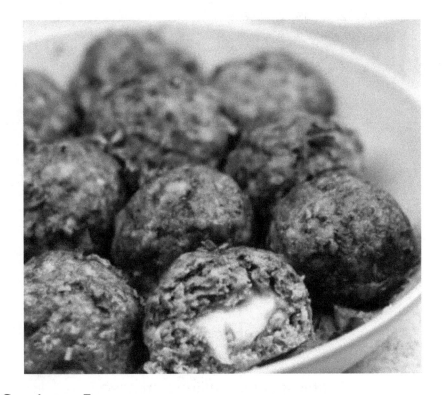

Servings: 5

Cooking Time: 25 Minutes

Ingredients:

- 2 eggs, beaten

- 1 pound ground pork

- 1/3 cup double cream

- 1 tablespoon fresh parsley

- Kosher salt and ground black pepper

- 1 teaspoon dried rosemary

- 10 (1-inch cubes of brie cheese

- 2 tablespoons scallions, minced

- 2 cloves garlic, minced

Directions:

1. Mix all ingredients, except for the brie cheese, until everything is well incorporated.

2. Roll the mixture into 10 patties; place a piece of cheese in the center of each patty and roll into a ball.

3. Roast in the preheated oven at 0 degrees F for about 20 minutes.

4. Storing

5. Place the meatballs in airtight containers or Ziploc bags; keep in your refrigerator for up to 3 to 4 days.

6. Freeze the meatballs in airtight containers or heavy-duty freezer bags. Freeze up to 3 to 4 months. To defrost, slowly reheat in a saucepan. Bon appétit!

Nutrition Info: 302 Calories; 13g Fat; 1.9g Carbs; 33.4g Protein; 0.3g Fiber

Spicy And Tangy Chicken Drumsticks

Servings: 6

Cooking Time: 55 Minutes

Ingredients:

- 3 chicken drumsticks, cut into chunks

- 1/2 stick butter

- 2 eggs

- 1/4 cup hemp seeds, ground

- Salt and cayenne pepper, to taste

- 2 tablespoons coconut aminos

- 3 teaspoons red wine vinegar

- 2 tablespoons salsa

- 2 cloves garlic, minced

Directions:

1. Rub the chicken with the butter, salt, and cayenne pepper.

2. Drizzle the chicken with the coconut aminos, vinegar, salsa, and garlic. Allow it to stand for 30 minutes in your refrigerator.

3. Whisk the eggs with the hemp seeds. Dip each chicken strip in the egg mixture. Place the chicken chunks in a parchment-lined baking pan.

4. Roast in the preheated oven at 390 degrees F for 25 minutes.

5. Storing

6. Divide the roasted chicken between airtight containers; keep in your refrigerator for up 3 to 4 days.

7. For freezing, place the roasted chicken in airtight containers or heavy-duty freezer bags. Freeze up to 3 months. Defrost in the refrigerator and reheat in a pan. Enjoy!

Nutrition Info: 420 Calories; 22g Fat; 5g Carbs; 35.3g Protein; 0.8g Fiber

Italian-style Chicken Meatballs With Parmesan

Servings: 6

Cooking Time: 20 Minutes

Ingredients:

- For the Meatballs:

- 1 ¼ pounds chicken, ground

- 1 tablespoon sage leaves, chopped

- 1 teaspoon shallot powder

- 1 teaspoon porcini powder

- 2 garlic cloves, finely minced

- 1/3 teaspoon dried basil

- 3/4 cup Parmesan cheese, grated

- 2 eggs, lightly beaten

- Salt and ground black pepper, to your liking

- 1/2 teaspoon cayenne pepper

- For the sauce:

- 2 tomatoes, pureed

- 1 cup chicken consommé

- 2 ½ tablespoons lard, room temperature

- 1 onion, peeled and finely chopped

Directions:

1. In a mixing bowl, combine all ingredients for the meatballs. Roll the mixture into bite-sized balls.

2. Melt 1 tablespoon of lard in a skillet over a moderately high heat. Sear the meatballs for about 3 minutes or until they are thoroughly cooked; reserve.

3. Melt the remaining lard and cook the onions until tender and translucent. Add in pureed tomatoes and chicken consommé and continue to cook for 4 minutes longer.

4. Add in the reserved meatballs, turn the heat to simmer and continue to cook for 6 to 7 minutes.

5. Storing

6. Place the meatballs in airtight containers or Ziploc bags; keep in your refrigerator for up to 3 to 4 days.

7. Freeze the meatballs in airtight containers or heavy-duty freezer bags. Freeze up to 3 to 4 months. To defrost, slowly reheat in a saucepan. Bon appétit!

Nutrition Info: 252 Calories; 9.7g Fat; 5.3g Carbs; 34.2g Protein; 1.4g Fiber

Sides & Appetizers Recipes

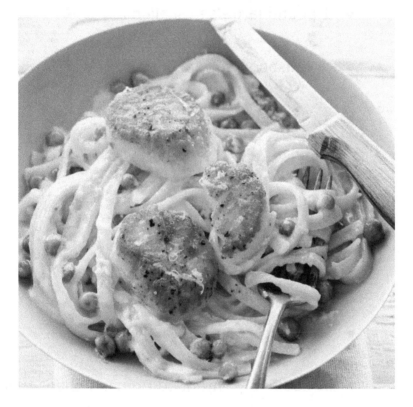

Servings: 5

Cooking Time: 15 Minutes

Ingredients:

- 8 ounces whole-wheat fettuccine (pasta, macaroni)

- 1 pound large sea scallops

- ¼ teaspoon salt, divided

- 1 tablespoon extra virgin olive oil

- 1 8-ounce bottle of clam juice

- 1 cup low-fat milk

- ¼ teaspoon ground white pepper

- 3 cups frozen peas, thawed

- ¾ cup finely shredded Romano cheese, divided

- 1/3 cup fresh chives, chopped

- ½ teaspoon freshly grated lemon zest

- 1 teaspoon lemon juice

Directions:

1. Boil water in a large pot and cook fettuccine according to package instructions.

2. Drain well and put it to the side.

3. Heat oil in a large, non-stick skillet over medium-high heat.

4. Pat the scallops dry and sprinkle them with 1/8 teaspoon of salt.

5. Add the scallops to the skillet and cook for about 2-3 minutes per side until golden brown. Remove scallops from pan.

6. Add clam juice to the pan you removed the scallops from.

7. In another bowl, whisk in milk, white pepper, flour, and remaining 1/8 teaspoon of salt.

8. Once the mixture is smooth, whisk into the pan with the clam juice.

9. Bring the entire mix to a simmer and keep stirring for about 1-2 minutes until the sauce is thick.

10. Return the scallops to the pan and add peas. Bring it to a simmer.

11. Stir in fettuccine, chives, ½ a cup of Romano cheese, lemon zest, and lemon juice.

12. Mix well until thoroughly combined.

13. Cool and spread over containers.

14. Before eating, serve with remaining cheese sprinkled on top.

15. Enjoy!

Nutrition Info:Per Serving: Calories: 388, Total Fat: 9.2 g, Saturated Fat: 3.7 g, Cholesterol: 33 mg, Sodium: 645 mg, Total Carbohydrate: 50.1 g, Dietary Fiber: 10.4 g, Total Sugars: 8.7 g, Protein: 24.9 g, Vitamin D: 25 mcg, Calcium: 293 mg, Iron: 4 mg, Potassium: 247 mg

Baked Mushrooms

Servings: 2

Cooking Time: 20 Minutes

Ingredients:

- ½ pound mushrooms (sliced)

- 2 tablespoons olive oil (onion and garlic flavored)

- 1 can tomatoes

- 1 cup Parmesan cheese

- ½ teaspoon oregano

- 1 tablespoon basil

- sea salt or plain salt

- freshly ground black pepper

Directions:

1. Heat the olive oil in the pan and add the mushrooms, salt, and pepper. Cook for about 2 minutes.

2. Then, transfer the mushrooms into a baking dish.

3. Now, in a separate bowl mix the tomatoes, basil, oregano, salt, and pepper, and layer it on the mushrooms. Top it with Parmesan cheese.

4. Finally, bake the dish at 0 degrees F for about 18-22 minutes or until done.

5. Serve warm.

Nutrition Info:Per Serving: Calories: 358, Total Fat: 27 g, Saturated Fat: 10.2 g, Cholesterol: 40 mg, Sodium: 535 mg, Total Carbohydrate: 13 g, Dietary Fiber: 3.5 g, Total Sugars: 6.7 g, Protein: 23.2 g, Vitamin D: 408 mcg, Calcium: 526 mg, Iron: 4 mg, Potassium: 797 mg

Mint Tabbouleh

Servings: 6

Cooking Time: 15 Minutes

Ingredients:

- ¼ cup fine bulgur

- 1/3 cup water, boiling

- 3 tablespoons lemon juice

- ¼ teaspoon honey

- 1 1/3 cups pistachios, finely chopped

- 1 cup curly parsley, finely chopped

- 1 small cucumber, finely chopped

- 1 medium tomato, finely chopped

- 4 green onions, finely chopped

- 1/3 cup fresh mint, finely chopped

- 3 tablespoons olive oil

Directions:

1. Take a large bowl and add bulgur and 3 cup of boiling water.

2. Allow it to stand for about 5 minutes.

3. Stir in honey and lemon juice and allow it to stand for 5 minutes more.

4. Fluff up the bulgur with a fork and stir in the rest of the Ingredients:.

5. Season with salt and pepper.

6. Enjoy!

Nutrition Info:Per Serving: Calories: 15 Total Fat: 13.5 g, Saturated Fat: 1.8 g, Cholesterol: 0 mg, Sodium: 78 mg, Total Carbohydrate: 9.2 g, Dietary Fiber: 2.8 g, Total Sugars: 2.9 g, Protein: 3.8 g,

Vitamin D: 0 mcg, Calcium: 46 mg, Iron: 2 mg, Potassium: 359 mg

Great Mediterranean Diet Recipes

Roasted Za'atar Salmon With Peppers And Sweet Potatoes

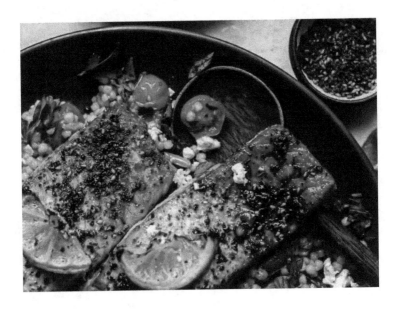

Servings: 4

Cooking Time: 25 Minutes

Ingredients:

- FOR THE VEGGIES

- 2 large red bell peppers, cut into ½-inch strips

- 1 pound sweet potatoes, peeled and cut into 1-inch chunks

- 1 tablespoon olive oil

- ¼ teaspoon kosher salt

- FOR THE SALMON

- 2¾ teaspoons sesame seeds

- 2¾ teaspoons dried thyme leaves

- 2¾ teaspoons sumac

- 1 pound skinless, boneless salmon fillet, divided into 4 pieces

- ⅛ teaspoon kosher salt

- 1 teaspoon olive oil

- 2 teaspoons freshly squeezed lemon juice

Directions:

1. TO MAKE THE VEGGIES

2. Preheat the oven to 4°F.

3. Place silicone baking mats or parchment paper on two sheet pans.

4. On the first pan, place the peppers and sweet potatoes. Pour the oil and sprinkle the salt over both and toss to coat. Spread everything out in an even layer. Place the sheet pan in the oven and set a timer for 10 minutes.

5. TO MAKE THE SALMON

6. Mix the sesame seeds, thyme, and sumac together in a small bowl to make the za'atar spice mix.

7. Place the salmon fillets on the second sheet pan. Sprinkle the salt evenly across the fillets. Spread ¼ teaspoon of oil and ½ teaspoon of lemon juice over each piece of salmon.

8. Pat 2 teaspoons of the za'atar spice mix over each piece of salmon.

9. When the veggie timer goes off, place the salmon in the oven with the veggies and bake for 10 minutes for salmon that is ½ inch thick and for 15 minutes for salmon that is 1 inch thick. The veggies should be done when the salmon is done cooking.

10. Place one quarter of the veggies and 1 piece of salmon in each of 4 separate containers.

11. STORAGE:Store covered containers in the refrigerator for up to 4 days.

Nutrition Info:Per Serving: Total calories: 295; Total fat: 10g; Saturated fat: 2g; Sodium: 249mg; Carbohydrates: 29g; Fiber: 6g; Protein: 25g

Conclusion

Here we are at the end of this wonderful journey. Did you enjoy yourselves? Keep learning to try and try again the recipes I have given you, you will see the benefits in the long run.

I always recommend talking to a nutritionist before starting any diet or nutritional plan.

Is your family happy? And the kids?

Follow me for more recipes.

Thank you

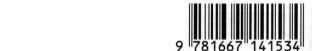